DR. BARBARA 21-DAY JUICING FOR CANCER CURE

Transform your health: join dr. Barbara's 21-days juicing journey to fight and defeat cancer naturally and reclaim vitality. Discover the power of nutrient-rich juices for healing and wellness

Edwardo Pedro

Table of Contents

COPYRIGHT © 2023

CHAPTER ONE

Introduction to Herbal Juicing and Cancer Treatment

Cancer, characterized by the abnormal growth of cells, remains one of the most challenging diseases to treat globally. Despite significant advancements in conventional cancer treatments like chemotherapy, radiation therapy, and surgery, their side effects and limitations have led many individuals to explore alternative and complementary therapies. Herbal juicing, a practice involving the extraction of juices from various herbs, fruits, and vegetables, has gained attention as a potential adjunctive therapy in cancer treatment.

Understanding Herbal Juicing

Herbal juicing involves the extraction of nutrient-rich juices from fresh herbs, fruits, and vegetables using a juicer or blender. Advocates of herbal juicing believe that consuming these juices can provide a concentrated source of vitamins, minerals, antioxidants, and phytochemicals, which may support overall health and potentially aid in disease prevention and management.

The Role of Herbal Juicing in Cancer Treatment

In the context of cancer treatment, herbal juicing is often explored as a complementary approach rather than a standalone therapy. Proponents suggest that certain herbs and plant-based foods contain compounds with anticancer properties, such as antioxidants, anti-inflammatory agents, and phytochemicals, which may help inhibit the growth of cancer cells, enhance immune function, and reduce the risk of cancer recurrence.

Popular Herbs and Ingredients in Cancer-Fighting Juices

Several herbs and ingredients are commonly used in cancer-fighting juices due to their purported health benefits and potential anticancer properties. These include:

1. **Turmeric**: Known for its active compound curcumin, turmeric possesses anti-inflammatory and antioxidant properties that may help combat cancer growth and reduce inflammation associated with cancer treatment.

2. **Ginger**: Ginger contains bioactive compounds like gingerol, which exhibit antioxidant and anti-inflammatory effects. It may help alleviate nausea and vomiting associated with chemotherapy and support digestive health during cancer treatment.

3. **Green Leafy Vegetables**: Kale, spinach, and other green leafy vegetables are rich sources of vitamins, minerals, and phytochemicals like chlorophyll and carotenoids, which have been studied for their potential anticancer effects.

4. **Cruciferous Vegetables**: Broccoli, cabbage, Brussels sprouts, and cauliflower are members of the cruciferous vegetable family, known for their high content of sulforaphane and other bioactive compounds that may help inhibit cancer cell growth and promote detoxification.

5. **Berries**: Blueberries, strawberries, raspberries, and other berries are rich in antioxidants like anthocyanins and flavonoids, which have been linked to reduced cancer risk and improved cellular health.

6. **Wheatgrass**: Wheatgrass juice is derived from the young shoots of the wheat plant and is praised for its high concentration of vitamins, minerals, enzymes, and chlorophyll. Some proponents believe it may help detoxify the body and boost immunity.

Evidence and Research

While anecdotal evidence and individual testimonials abound regarding the benefits of herbal juicing in cancer treatment, scientific research on the topic is still limited. Most studies investigating the anticancer properties of herbs and plant-based foods have been conducted in laboratory settings or animal models, with relatively few human clinical trials.

However, some preliminary research suggests that certain compounds found in herbs and plant foods may indeed exhibit anticancer effects. For example, studies on curcumin, the active compound in turmeric, have shown promising results in terms of its ability to inhibit cancer cell proliferation, induce apoptosis (cell death), and modulate signaling pathways involved in cancer development and progression.

Similarly, research on ginger has demonstrated its potential to suppress tumor growth, enhance the efficacy of chemotherapy and radiation therapy, and mitigate treatment-related side effects like nausea and vomiting. However, more high-quality clinical trials are needed to validate these findings and determine the optimal dosages and formulations for cancer patients.

Safety Considerations and Potential Risks

While herbal juicing is generally considered safe for most individuals when consumed as part of a balanced diet, there are some important safety considerations and potential risks to be aware of, especially for cancer patients undergoing treatment. These include:

1. **Interactions with Medications**: Some herbs and plant-based foods used in juicing may interact with certain medications commonly prescribed in cancer treatment, affecting their

efficacy or causing adverse effects. It's essential for cancer patients to consult with their healthcare providers before incorporating herbal juices into their regimen, especially if they're taking medications like chemotherapy drugs or blood thinners.

2. **Nutrient Imbalances**: Drinking large quantities of herbal juices without proper guidance can lead to nutrient imbalances or deficiencies, particularly if they're consumed as meal replacements rather than supplements. Cancer patients should aim for a varied and nutrient-rich diet that includes a combination of whole foods, herbal juices, and other beverages to ensure adequate intake of essential nutrients.

3. **Contamination and Food Safety**: Raw fruits, vegetables, and herbs used in juicing may carry bacteria, pesticides, or other contaminants that can pose health risks, especially for individuals with weakened immune systems due to cancer or its treatment. It's essential to wash produce thoroughly and choose organic options whenever possible to minimize exposure to harmful substances.

4. **Digestive Issues**: Some cancer patients may experience digestive issues like diarrhea, constipation, or gastrointestinal discomfort, which can be exacerbated by certain ingredients in herbal juices, such as high-fiber

vegetables or acidic fruits. Adjusting the ingredients and quantities based on individual tolerance levels may help alleviate these symptoms.

Conclusion

Herbal juicing is a popular practice among individuals seeking natural and holistic approaches to cancer treatment and prevention. While it's not a substitute for conventional medical therapies, herbal juices may complement standard treatments by providing essential nutrients, antioxidants, and bioactive compounds that support overall health and well-being.

However, more research is needed to better understand the specific effects of herbal juicing on cancer prevention, treatment outcomes, and safety profiles. Cancer patients should consult with their healthcare providers before incorporating herbal juices into their regimen to ensure they're receiving evidence-based recommendations tailored to their individual needs and medical history.

CHAPTER TWO

Understanding Cancer: Types, Causes, and Treatment Options

Cancer is a complex group of diseases characterized by the abnormal growth and spread of cells in the body. It can develop in virtually any tissue or organ and has the potential to invade nearby tissues and metastasize to distant sites. Understanding the various types of cancer, their underlying causes, and available treatment options is essential for effective prevention, diagnosis, and management of this widespread disease.

Types of Cancer

Cancer can arise in different parts of the body and is classified based on the type of cells where it originates. Some common types of cancer include:

1. **Carcinomas**: These cancers develop from epithelial cells, which line the surfaces of organs and tissues. Carcinomas are the most common type of cancer and can occur in the skin, lungs, breast, colon, prostate, and other organs.

2. **Sarcomas**: Sarcomas originate in the body's connective tissues, including bones, muscles, cartilage, and blood vessels. Examples of sarcomas include osteosarcoma (bone cancer) and leiomyosarcoma (muscle cancer).

3. **Leukemias**: Leukemias are cancers of the blood-forming tissues, such as the bone marrow and lymphatic system. They involve the overproduction of abnormal white blood cells, which can interfere with normal blood cell production and function.

4. **Lymphomas**: Lymphomas affect the lymphatic system, which plays a crucial role in the body's immune response. They arise from lymphocytes, a type of white blood cell, and can occur in lymph nodes, spleen, bone marrow, and other lymphoid tissues.

5. **Central Nervous System (CNS) Tumors**: These tumors develop in the brain or spinal cord and can be benign (non-cancerous) or malignant (cancerous). Examples include gliomas, meningiomas, and medulloblastomas.

6. **Melanomas**: Melanomas are cancers that originate in melanocytes, the pigment-producing cells responsible for skin coloration. They typically develop in the skin but can also occur in the eyes and mucous membranes.

Causes of Cancer

Cancer is a multifactorial disease influenced by a combination of genetic, environmental, and lifestyle factors. While the exact cause of cancer can vary depending on the type and individual circumstances, some common risk factors include:

1. **Genetic Mutations**: Mutations in certain genes can increase the risk of cancer by disrupting normal cell growth and division. These mutations may be inherited from parents or acquired over time due to environmental exposures or lifestyle choices.

2. **Environmental Exposures**: Exposure to carcinogenic substances in the environment, such as tobacco smoke, air pollution, ultraviolet (UV) radiation, asbestos, and industrial chemicals, can increase the risk of developing cancer.

3. **Lifestyle Factors**: Unhealthy lifestyle choices, such as smoking, excessive alcohol consumption, poor diet, lack of physical activity, and obesity, are associated with an increased risk of several types of cancer.

4. **Age**: The risk of cancer tends to increase with age, as cellular damage accumulates over time, and the body's ability to repair damaged DNA declines.

5. **Hormonal Factors**: Hormonal imbalances or changes in hormone levels can contribute to the development of certain cancers, such as breast, ovarian, and prostate cancer.

6. **Family History**: A family history of cancer can indicate an inherited predisposition to the disease, although most cases of cancer are not directly linked to genetics.

Treatment Options for Cancer

The treatment approach for cancer depends on various factors, including the type and stage of the disease, the patient's overall health, and individual preferences. Common treatment modalities include:

1. **Surgery**: Surgical removal of cancerous tumors is often used to treat localized cancers that have not spread to other parts of the body. It may be performed alone or in combination with other treatments.

2. **Chemotherapy**: Chemotherapy involves the use of drugs to kill cancer cells or slow their growth. It can be administered orally, intravenously, or topically and is often used in combination with surgery, radiation therapy, or other treatments.

3. **Radiation Therapy**: Radiation therapy uses high-energy radiation to destroy cancer cells and shrink tumors. It can be delivered externally (external beam radiation) or internally (brachytherapy) and may be used as a primary treatment or in conjunction with surgery or chemotherapy.

4. **Immunotherapy**: Immunotherapy harnesses the body's immune system to recognize and attack cancer cells. It includes various approaches such as checkpoint inhibitors, adoptive cell therapy, and cancer vaccines.

5. **Targeted Therapy**: Targeted therapy drugs are designed to specifically target cancer cells by interfering with specific molecules involved in cancer growth and progression. They may be used alone or in combination with other treatments.

6. **Hormone Therapy**: Hormone therapy is used to block or suppress the production of hormones that fuel certain types of cancer, such as breast and prostate cancer. It may involve medications or surgical removal of hormone-producing organs.

7. **Stem Cell Transplantation**: Stem cell transplantation, also known as bone marrow or hematopoietic stem cell transplantation, may be used to treat certain blood cancers like leukemia, lymphoma, and multiple myeloma. It involves replacing diseased or damaged bone marrow with healthy stem cells.

Conclusion

Cancer is a complex and heterogeneous disease with multiple types, causes, and treatment options. Understanding the underlying mechanisms of cancer development, as well as the various factors that contribute to its onset and progression, is crucial for developing effective prevention strategies and personalized treatment approaches. By combining advances in research, technology, and clinical care, efforts to combat cancer continue to evolve, offering hope for improved outcomes and quality of life for patients affected by this devastating illness.

CHAPTER THREE

The Role of Nutrition in Cancer Prevention and Healing

Nutrition plays a fundamental role in cancer prevention and healing, influencing various aspects of the disease's development, progression, and treatment outcomes. A growing body of research suggests that adopting a healthy and balanced diet rich in nutrient-dense foods can help reduce the risk of cancer and support the body's natural defenses against the disease. Additionally, nutrition plays a crucial role in supporting individuals undergoing cancer treatment, helping to manage symptoms, maintain strength and energy levels, and enhance overall well-being.

Nutritional Factors in Cancer Prevention

1. **Antioxidants**: Antioxidants are compounds that help neutralize harmful free radicals in the body, which can damage cells and contribute to cancer development. Foods rich in antioxidants, such as fruits, vegetables, nuts, seeds, and whole grains, are essential components of a cancer-preventive diet.

2. **Fiber**: A high-fiber diet, primarily derived from fruits, vegetables, legumes, and whole grains, has been associated with a reduced risk of certain cancers, including colorectal

cancer. Fiber helps promote regular bowel movements, which can aid in the elimination of toxins and carcinogens from the body.

3. **Healthy Fats**: Consuming healthy fats, such as those found in avocados, nuts, seeds, and fatty fish like salmon, can help reduce inflammation and support overall health. Omega-3 fatty acids, in particular, have been shown to have anti-inflammatory properties and may help lower the risk of certain cancers.

4. **Cruciferous Vegetables**: Vegetables from the cruciferous family, such as broccoli, cauliflower, Brussels sprouts, and kale, contain compounds like sulforaphane and indole-3-carbinol, which have been linked to a reduced risk of cancer. These vegetables may help inhibit cancer cell growth and promote detoxification pathways in the body.

5. **Herbs and Spices**: Certain herbs and spices, including turmeric, ginger, garlic, and cinnamon, contain bioactive compounds with anti-inflammatory and antioxidant properties that may help protect against cancer. Incorporating these herbs and spices into the diet can add flavor and nutritional benefits.

6. **Limiting Processed Foods and Sugars**: Diets high in processed foods, sugary beverages, refined carbohydrates, and red or processed meats have been associated with an

increased risk of cancer. Limiting intake of these foods and opting for whole, unprocessed foods can help reduce cancer risk and promote overall health.

Nutrition During Cancer Treatment

1. **Maintaining Nutritional Status**: Cancer treatment, such as chemotherapy, radiation therapy, and surgery, can place significant demands on the body and may lead to side effects like nausea, vomiting, loss of appetite, and weight loss. It's essential for cancer patients to maintain adequate nutritional intake to support their immune function, strength, and energy levels during treatment.

2. **Individualized Nutrition Plans**: Cancer patients may benefit from working with registered dietitians or nutritionists to develop personalized nutrition plans tailored to their specific needs and treatment goals. These plans may include strategies to manage treatment-related side effects, ensure adequate nutrient intake, and maintain hydration and energy levels.

3. **Emphasis on Protein and Calories**: Adequate protein and calorie intake are essential for supporting muscle mass, immune function, and overall recovery during cancer treatment. Foods rich in protein, such as lean meats, poultry, fish, eggs, dairy products, legumes, and nuts, should be prioritized to meet these needs.

4. **Hydration**: Staying hydrated is crucial for cancer patients, especially those experiencing side effects like nausea, vomiting, diarrhea, or mouth sores. Drinking plenty of fluids, including water, herbal teas, broths, and electrolyte-replenishing beverages, can help prevent dehydration and support overall well-being.

5. **Supplementation**: In some cases, cancer patients may require nutritional supplementation to address specific nutrient deficiencies or support treatment-related side effects. Supplements such as vitamin D, B vitamins, omega-3 fatty acids, and probiotics may be recommended under the guidance of healthcare providers.

Conclusion

Nutrition plays a vital role in both cancer prevention and healing, influencing various aspects of the disease's development, progression, and treatment outcomes. Adopting a healthy and balanced diet rich in nutrient-dense foods, including fruits, vegetables, whole grains, lean proteins, and healthy fats, can help reduce the risk of cancer and support overall health and well-being. Additionally, personalized nutrition plans tailored to the individual needs of cancer patients can help manage treatment-related side effects, maintain nutritional status, and optimize recovery. By emphasizing the importance of nutrition as part of comprehensive cancer care, healthcare providers can empower patients to take an active role in their health and well-being throughout the cancer journey.

CHAPTER FOUR

Introduction to Dr. Barbara's 21-Day Herbal Juicing Protocol

Dr. Barbara's 21-Day Herbal Juicing Protocol is a comprehensive program designed to promote health, vitality, and well-being through the power of herbal juicing. Developed by renowned herbalist and wellness expert, Dr. Barbara, this protocol offers a structured approach to incorporating herbal juices into daily life, with the aim of detoxifying the body, boosting immunity, and supporting overall health.

Understanding Herbal Juicing

Herbal juicing involves the extraction of nutrient-rich juices from fresh herbs, fruits, and vegetables using a juicer or blender. Unlike traditional juicing methods that focus solely on fruits and vegetables, Dr. Barbara's protocol emphasizes the inclusion of specific herbs known for their therapeutic properties and health benefits. By harnessing the healing properties of herbs, this protocol aims to enhance the nutritional value and therapeutic efficacy of the juices, providing a natural and holistic approach to wellness.

The Principles of Dr. Barbara's Protocol

Dr. Barbara's 21-Day Herbal Juicing Protocol is based on several key principles:

1. **Detoxification**: The protocol is designed to support the body's natural detoxification processes, helping to eliminate toxins, waste products, and accumulated metabolic byproducts that may impair cellular function and contribute to health issues.

2. **Nutrient Replenishment**: Herbal juices are rich sources of vitamins, minerals, antioxidants, and phytonutrients that nourish the body at the cellular level, supporting optimal health and vitality.

3. **Immune Support**: Many of the herbs included in the protocol have immune-modulating properties, helping to strengthen the body's defenses against infections, pathogens, and environmental stressors.

4. **Inflammation Reduction**: Chronic inflammation is a common underlying factor in many chronic diseases, including cancer, heart disease, and autoimmune conditions. The anti-inflammatory properties of certain herbs can help reduce inflammation and promote healing throughout the body.

5. **Gut Health**: The protocol prioritizes gut health, recognizing the importance of a healthy microbiome in supporting digestion, nutrient absorption, immune function, and overall well-being. Certain herbs included in the protocol may help promote a balanced gut microbiota and support digestive health.

Key Components of the Protocol

Dr. Barbara's 21-Day Herbal Juicing Protocol consists of several key components:

1. **Herbal Juice Recipes**: The protocol provides a variety of herbal juice recipes formulated by Dr. Barbara, each carefully crafted to deliver specific health benefits. These recipes combine a blend of fresh fruits, vegetables, and herbs, with an emphasis on organic and locally sourced ingredients whenever possible.

2. **Daily Juicing Schedule**: Participants are encouraged to follow a daily juicing schedule, incorporating herbal juices into their morning routine, snacks, or meals throughout the day. Consistency is key to experiencing the full benefits of the protocol.

3. **Supplemental Recommendations**: In addition to herbal juices, Dr. Barbara may recommend specific dietary supplements, herbal tinctures, or botanical extracts to support individual health goals and address specific health concerns.

4. **Lifestyle Guidelines**: The protocol may include lifestyle recommendations such as stress management techniques, exercise, sleep hygiene, and mindfulness practices to promote holistic wellness and enhance the effectiveness of the juicing protocol.

Conclusion

Dr. Barbara's 21-Day Herbal Juicing Protocol offers a structured and holistic approach to improving health and well-being through the power of herbal juicing. By incorporating nutrient-rich herbal juices into daily life and following the principles of detoxification, immune support, inflammation reduction, and gut health, participants can experience enhanced vitality, increased energy, and improved overall health. With its emphasis on natural, whole-food ingredients and personalized wellness strategies, this protocol serves as a valuable tool for individuals seeking to optimize their health and embark on a journey towards wellness and vitality.

CHAPTER FIVE

Selecting the right herbs for cancer healing

Selecting the right herbs for cancer healing is a crucial aspect of integrative and complementary cancer care. While herbs are not a substitute for conventional cancer treatments such as chemotherapy, radiation therapy, and surgery, they can complement medical interventions and support overall health and well-being. When choosing herbs for cancer healing, several factors should be considered, including the herb's potential anticancer properties, safety profile, compatibility with other treatments, and individual health needs and preferences.

1. Anticancer Properties: When selecting herbs for cancer healing, it's essential to choose those with documented or potential anticancer properties. Numerous herbs contain bioactive compounds that have been studied for their ability to inhibit cancer cell growth, induce apoptosis (cell death), reduce inflammation, and enhance immune function. Examples of herbs with potential anticancer properties include turmeric, ginger, green tea, garlic, echinacea, and astragalus.

2. Safety Profile: Safety is paramount when using herbs for cancer healing, especially in individuals undergoing conventional cancer treatments. Some herbs may interact with medications or exacerbate treatment-related side effects, while others may be contraindicated in certain medical conditions. It's crucial to consult with a qualified healthcare provider, such as a naturopathic doctor or herbalist, before incorporating herbs into a cancer treatment regimen. Additionally, it's essential to use herbs from reputable sources, preferably organic and free from contaminants.

3. Compatibility with Conventional Treatments: Herbs selected for cancer healing should be compatible with conventional cancer treatments to ensure synergy and minimize the risk of adverse interactions. Some herbs may enhance the effectiveness of chemotherapy or radiation therapy, while others may interfere with treatment efficacy or increase the risk of side effects. Healthcare providers knowledgeable in integrative oncology can provide guidance on herb-drug interactions and help tailor a personalized treatment plan that integrates herbs with conventional cancer therapies.

4. Individual Health Needs and Preferences: The selection of herbs for cancer healing should take into account the individual's health needs, preferences, and treatment goals. For example, some individuals may prefer herbs with adaptogenic properties to help manage stress and support adrenal function during cancer treatment, while others may focus on herbs with immune-stimulating or anti-inflammatory properties to enhance overall immune function and reduce treatment-related inflammation. Additionally, herbs may be selected based on specific symptoms or side effects experienced during cancer treatment, such as nausea, fatigue, pain, or digestive issues.

5. Evidence-Based Research: While traditional wisdom and anecdotal evidence may inform the selection of herbs for cancer healing, it's essential to prioritize herbs with evidence-based research supporting their efficacy and safety in the context of cancer care. Clinical studies, preclinical research, and systematic reviews can provide valuable insights into the potential benefits and limitations of specific herbs for cancer prevention, treatment, and symptom management.

Conclusion

Selecting the right herbs for cancer healing requires careful consideration of the herb's potential anticancer properties, safety profile, compatibility with conventional treatments, individual health needs, and evidence-based research. By working closely with qualified healthcare providers knowledgeable in integrative oncology, individuals can develop personalized treatment plans that incorporate herbs as part of a comprehensive approach to cancer care. With proper guidance and supervision, herbs can serve as valuable allies in supporting overall health, well-being, and resilience throughout the cancer journey.

CHAPTER SIX

Juicing recipes for boosting immunity and detoxification

Juicing recipes for boosting immunity and detoxification can incorporate a variety of nutrient-rich fruits, vegetables, and herbs known for their immune-supportive and detoxifying properties. These recipes aim to provide a concentrated source of vitamins, minerals, antioxidants, and phytonutrients that promote overall health and well-being. Here are two juicing recipes designed to support immunity and detoxification:

1. Immune-Boosting Green Juice:

Ingredients:

- 2 cups spinach
- 1 cucumber
- 2 stalks celery
- 1 green apple
- 1 inch piece of ginger
- 1 lemon (peeled)
- 1 handful of fresh parsley

Instructions:

1. Wash all the ingredients thoroughly.

2. Chop the cucumber, celery, and apple into smaller pieces for easier juicing.

3. Peel the lemon and ginger.

4. Juice all the ingredients using a juicer.

5. Stir the juice well to combine the flavors.

6. Pour the juice into a glass and serve immediately.

Benefits:

- Spinach is rich in vitamins A, C, and K, as well as iron and antioxidants, which support immune function and overall health.

- Cucumber and celery are hydrating vegetables that provide electrolytes and micronutrients essential for detoxification and cellular function.

- Green apple adds sweetness and fiber, while also providing vitamin C and antioxidants.

- Ginger has anti-inflammatory and immune-boosting properties, making it beneficial for supporting immune health and reducing inflammation.

- Lemon provides vitamin C and citric acid, which help alkalize the body and support detoxification pathways.

- Parsley is rich in chlorophyll and antioxidants, which aid in detoxification and promote overall health.

2. Citrus Carrot Detox Juice:

Ingredients:

- 4 carrots

- 2 oranges (peeled)

- 1 lemon (peeled)

- 1 inch piece of turmeric root

- 1 inch piece of ginger

Instructions:

1. Wash all the ingredients thoroughly.

2. Peel the oranges and lemon.

3. Chop the carrots, oranges, and lemon into smaller pieces for easier juicing.

4. Peel the turmeric root and ginger.

5. Juice all the ingredients using a juicer.

6. Stir the juice well to combine the flavors.

7. Pour the juice into a glass and serve immediately.

Benefits:

- Carrots are rich in beta-carotene, vitamin A, and antioxidants, which support liver function and promote detoxification.

- Oranges and lemon provide vitamin C, which boosts immune function and supports collagen production.

- Turmeric root contains curcumin, a potent anti-inflammatory compound that supports liver health and detoxification pathways.

- Ginger aids digestion, reduces inflammation, and supports immune function, making it beneficial for detoxification and overall health.

Note: These juicing recipes are intended to complement a healthy and balanced diet, not replace it. It's essential to consume a variety of fruits, vegetables, whole grains, lean proteins, and healthy fats to support overall health and well-being. Additionally, individuals with specific health conditions or dietary restrictions should consult with a healthcare provider or registered dietitian before making significant changes to their diet or incorporating new foods or supplements.

CHAPTER SEVEN

HERBAL JUICES FOR CANCER PATIENTS

Herbal juices can be a valuable addition to a cancer patient's diet, offering natural compounds that may help alleviate common symptoms associated with the disease and its treatment. While herbal juices are not a substitute for medical treatment, they can complement conventional therapies and provide relief from symptoms such as nausea, fatigue, digestive issues, and immune suppression. Here are some herbal juice recipes specifically formulated to alleviate common cancer symptoms:

1. Ginger-Lemon Soother:

Ingredients:

- 1-2 inches of fresh ginger root

- 1 lemon (peeled)

- 1-2 tablespoons of honey (optional)

- 1-2 cups of water or coconut water

Instructions:

1. Peel and chop the ginger root into smaller pieces.

2. Peel the lemon.

3. Juice the ginger and lemon using a juicer.

4. Dilute the juice with water or coconut water to taste.

5. Add honey if desired for sweetness.

6. Stir well and serve chilled or over ice.

Benefits:

- Ginger has anti-nausea properties and can help alleviate chemotherapy-induced nausea and vomiting.

- Lemon provides vitamin C and antioxidants, which support immune function and help combat fatigue.

- Honey adds sweetness and may soothe a sore throat or dry mouth common during cancer treatment.

- Coconut water provides electrolytes and hydration, which is essential for managing fatigue and promoting overall well-being.

2. Turmeric-Apple Digestive Tonic:

Ingredients:

- 1-2 inches of fresh turmeric root (or 1-2 teaspoons of ground turmeric)

- 2 apples (cored and chopped)

- 1 cucumber

- 1-2 stalks of celery

- 1 inch piece of ginger

- 1 lemon (peeled)

Instructions:

1. Peel and chop the turmeric root (if using fresh).

2. Core and chop the apples.

3. Wash the cucumber and celery.

4. Peel the lemon.

5. Juice all the ingredients using a juicer.

6. Stir well and serve immediately.

Benefits:

- Turmeric contains curcumin, a powerful anti-inflammatory compound that may help alleviate inflammation and digestive discomfort associated with cancer treatment.

- Apples provide fiber and antioxidants, which support digestive health and help regulate bowel movements.

- Cucumber and celery are hydrating vegetables that promote hydration and provide essential nutrients for overall health and well-being.

- Ginger aids digestion, reduces bloating, and may help alleviate nausea and gastrointestinal symptoms.

3. Mint-Berry Immune Booster:

Ingredients:

- 1 cup of mixed berries (such as strawberries, blueberries, raspberries)
- 1 handful of fresh mint leaves
- 1 cucumber
- 1-2 cups of coconut water or water

Instructions:

1. Wash the berries and mint leaves.

2. Wash the cucumber.

3. Juice the berries, mint leaves, and cucumber using a juicer.

4. Dilute the juice with coconut water or water to taste.

5. Stir well and serve chilled.

Benefits:

- Berries are rich in antioxidants, vitamins, and minerals that support immune function and overall health.
- Mint has soothing properties and may help alleviate digestive discomfort, bloating, and nausea.

- Cucumber provides hydration and essential nutrients while adding a refreshing flavor to the juice.

- Coconut water replenishes electrolytes and provides hydration, which is crucial for managing fatigue and promoting well-being during cancer treatment.

Note: These herbal juice recipes are intended to complement conventional cancer treatments and provide relief from common symptoms associated with the disease and its treatment. It's essential for cancer patients to consult with their healthcare providers before incorporating herbal juices into their diet, especially if they're taking medications or undergoing treatment. Additionally, individuals with specific dietary restrictions or allergies should modify recipes accordingly or consult with a registered dietitian for personalized recommendations.

CHAPTER EIGHT

Implementing a holistic approach to cancer healing

Implementing a holistic approach to cancer healing involves addressing the physical, emotional, mental, and spiritual aspects of the individual, with the goal of promoting overall well-being and supporting the body's innate healing mechanisms. This approach recognizes that cancer affects the whole person and involves various interconnected factors that contribute to health and disease. Here are key components of a holistic approach to cancer healing:

1. Nutritional Support:

- Emphasize a whole-foods, plant-based diet rich in fruits, vegetables, whole grains, legumes, nuts, and seeds, which provide essential nutrients, antioxidants, and phytonutrients that support immune function and overall health.

- Incorporate herbal remedies, supplements, and therapeutic foods known for their anti-inflammatory, immune-boosting, and detoxifying properties, such as turmeric, ginger, garlic, green tea, and cruciferous vegetables.

- Work with a registered dietitian or nutritionist knowledgeable in oncology to develop a personalized nutrition plan tailored to individual needs, treatment goals, and dietary preferences.

2. Physical Well-being:

- Encourage regular physical activity, such as walking, yoga, tai chi, or gentle stretching exercises, to improve circulation, reduce stress, and enhance overall vitality.

- Explore complementary therapies and integrative modalities that support physical healing and symptom management, such as acupuncture, massage therapy, chiropractic care, and energy healing techniques.

- Prioritize rest and relaxation, ensuring adequate sleep, stress management, and self-care practices to promote healing and resilience.

3. Emotional and Mental Health:

- Provide psychosocial support and counseling services to address the emotional and psychological impact of cancer diagnosis and treatment, including anxiety, depression, fear, grief, and existential concerns.

- Encourage expressive therapies, such as art therapy, music therapy, journaling, or mindfulness meditation, as creative outlets for emotional expression, self-reflection, and coping with stress.

- Foster a supportive community and social network of family, friends, support groups, and healthcare providers who can offer empathy, understanding, and encouragement throughout the cancer journey.

4. Spiritual and Existential Care:

- Support spiritual exploration and existential reflection, helping individuals find meaning, purpose, and connection amidst the challenges of cancer.

- Offer opportunities for spiritual practices, rituals, prayer, meditation, or contemplative exercises that nurture the soul, deepen self-awareness, and cultivate inner peace and resilience.

- Respect individual beliefs, values, and cultural traditions, honoring diverse spiritual perspectives and providing a compassionate presence that acknowledges the sacredness of life and the mystery of suffering.

5. Integrative Cancer Care:

- Collaborate with a multidisciplinary team of healthcare providers, including oncologists, integrative medicine specialists, naturopathic doctors, nurses, therapists, and holistic practitioners, to provide comprehensive and coordinated care.

- Individualize treatment plans based on the unique needs, preferences, and goals of each patient, integrating conventional medical therapies with complementary and alternative modalities as appropriate.

- Foster open communication, shared decision-making, and patient empowerment, empowering individuals to play an active role in their healing journey and make informed choices about their care.

Conclusion: A holistic approach to cancer healing embraces the interconnectedness of body, mind, and spirit, recognizing that each aspect of the individual contributes to health and well-being. By addressing physical, emotional, mental, and spiritual needs through nutrition, physical activity, emotional support, spiritual care, and integrative therapies, individuals can experience greater resilience, vitality, and quality of life throughout the cancer journey. Collaborative and compassionate care that honors the whole person is essential for promoting healing, fostering hope, and restoring wholeness amidst the challenges of cancer.

CHAPTER NINE

Lifestyle modifications

Lifestyle modifications play a crucial role in supporting the healing process for individuals dealing with cancer. These changes aim to optimize overall health and well-being, enhance treatment outcomes, reduce the risk of cancer recurrence, and improve quality of life. Here are several lifestyle modifications that can support the healing process:

1. Nutrition and Diet:

- Adopt a balanced and nutrient-rich diet that emphasizes whole foods, including fruits, vegetables, whole grains, lean proteins, and healthy fats.

- Limit processed foods, sugary beverages, refined carbohydrates, and red or processed meats, which may contribute to inflammation and increase cancer risk.

- Stay hydrated by drinking plenty of water throughout the day, and limit alcohol consumption, which can impair immune function and interfere with healing.

- Consider incorporating specific foods and dietary supplements known for their anti-inflammatory, immune-boosting, and detoxifying properties, such as turmeric, ginger, garlic, green tea, and omega-3 fatty acids.

2. Physical Activity and Exercise:

- Engage in regular physical activity, such as walking, swimming, cycling, yoga, or strength training, to improve circulation, strengthen muscles, boost immune function, and enhance overall well-being.

- Aim for at least 150 minutes of moderate-intensity aerobic exercise or 75 minutes of vigorous-intensity exercise per week, as recommended by the American Cancer Society.

- Listen to your body and adjust the intensity and duration of exercise based on energy levels, treatment side effects, and individual preferences.

- Incorporate relaxation techniques, such as deep breathing, meditation, tai chi, or guided imagery, to reduce stress, promote relaxation, and support the body's natural healing processes.

3. Stress Management and Mindfulness:

- Practice stress reduction techniques, such as mindfulness meditation, progressive muscle relaxation, or biofeedback, to lower stress hormone levels, reduce inflammation, and promote healing.

- Prioritize self-care activities that bring joy and relaxation, such as spending time in nature, engaging in hobbies, listening to music, or connecting with loved ones.

- Seek emotional support from family, friends, support groups, or mental health professionals to process feelings of anxiety, depression, fear, or grief related to cancer diagnosis and treatment.

- Cultivate a positive mindset and resilience by focusing on gratitude, hope, and meaningful activities that inspire a sense of purpose and well-being.

4. Sleep Hygiene and Restorative Rest:

- Establish a regular sleep schedule and create a relaxing bedtime routine to promote restful sleep and optimize circadian rhythms.

- Create a comfortable sleep environment that is cool, dark, quiet, and free from electronic devices that may disrupt sleep.

- Practice good sleep hygiene habits, such as avoiding caffeine and stimulating activities before bedtime, limiting screen time, and practicing relaxation techniques to prepare the body for sleep.

- Listen to your body and prioritize rest and recovery as needed, allowing time for relaxation, naps, and downtime to recharge and restore energy levels.

5. Tobacco Cessation and Substance Use Reduction:

- Quit smoking and avoid exposure to secondhand smoke, as tobacco use is a significant risk factor for cancer development, recurrence, and treatment-related complications.

- Limit or avoid alcohol consumption, as excessive drinking can weaken the immune system, interfere with treatment efficacy, and increase the risk of cancer recurrence.

- Seek support from healthcare providers, counselors, or smoking cessation programs to quit smoking or reduce substance use and address any underlying addiction issues.

6. Regular Medical Check-Ups and Follow-Up Care:

- Attend scheduled medical appointments and follow-up visits with healthcare providers, including oncologists, primary care physicians, and specialists, to monitor treatment progress, address any concerns, and adjust treatment plans as needed.

- Participate in recommended cancer screening tests and surveillance programs to detect cancer recurrence or new cancerous growths at an early stage when treatment is most effective.

- Stay informed about the latest advancements in cancer treatment and supportive care, and advocate for your health by asking questions, seeking second opinions, and staying actively involved in decision-making about your care.

Conclusion: By making lifestyle modifications that prioritize nutrition, physical activity, stress management, sleep hygiene, tobacco cessation, and regular medical follow-up, individuals can support the healing process, optimize treatment outcomes, and improve overall quality of life during and after cancer treatment. These changes empower individuals to take an active role in their health and well-being, fostering resilience, hope, and a sense of empowerment throughout the cancer journey.

CHAPTER TEN

Monitoring progress and maintaining long-term health after completing a 21-day program

Monitoring progress and maintaining long-term health after completing a 21-day program requires a comprehensive approach that encompasses ongoing self-assessment, lifestyle modifications, and supportive strategies to sustain positive changes and promote overall well-being. Here are some key steps to monitor progress and maintain long-term health after completing the program:

1. Regular Self-Assessment:

- Continuously monitor your physical, emotional, and mental well-being to gauge progress and identify areas for improvement.

- Keep track of symptoms, energy levels, mood, sleep quality, and overall health using a journal, diary, or health tracking app.

- Reflect on your experiences during the program, noting any changes in dietary habits, physical activity, stress levels, and coping strategies.

2. Healthy Lifestyle Habits:

- Maintain healthy eating habits by continuing to prioritize nutrient-rich foods, such as fruits, vegetables, whole grains, lean proteins, and healthy fats.

- Incorporate regular physical activity into your daily routine, aiming for at least 150 minutes of moderate-intensity aerobic exercise per week, as recommended by health guidelines.

- Practice stress management techniques, relaxation exercises, and mindfulness practices to reduce stress, promote relaxation, and support overall well-being.

- Prioritize restorative sleep by establishing a consistent sleep schedule, creating a relaxing bedtime routine, and optimizing sleep environment.

3. Long-Term Dietary Changes:

- Gradually integrate the lessons learned from the 21-day program into your long-term dietary habits, incorporating more plant-based foods, whole grains, and healthy fats into your meals.

- Experiment with new recipes, flavors, and cooking techniques to keep meals interesting and enjoyable, while still prioritizing nutrient density and healthful ingredients.

- Stay hydrated by drinking plenty of water throughout the day and limiting intake of sugary beverages, alcohol, and caffeinated drinks.

4. Mindful Eating Practices:

- Practice mindful eating techniques, such as slowing down during meals, savoring each bite, and paying attention to hunger and fullness cues.

- Listen to your body's signals and eat intuitively, choosing foods that nourish and energize you while avoiding those that make you feel sluggish or unwell.

- Stay attuned to emotional triggers for eating, such as stress, boredom, or anxiety, and find alternative ways to cope with emotions without resorting to food.

5. Continued Education and Support:

- Stay informed about nutrition, health, and wellness topics by reading books, attending workshops, or following reputable sources of information online.

- Seek ongoing support from healthcare providers, nutritionists, dietitians, or support groups to address any challenges or questions related to maintaining a healthy lifestyle.

- Connect with others who share similar health goals and experiences, whether through online communities, social networks, or local support groups.

6. Regular Health Check-Ups:

- Schedule regular health check-ups and screenings with your healthcare provider to monitor your overall health, track progress, and address any potential health concerns or risk factors.

- Discuss any changes in symptoms, lifestyle habits, or treatment plans with your healthcare provider, and collaborate on strategies to optimize your long-term health and well-being.

Conclusion: Maintaining long-term health after completing a 21-day program requires ongoing commitment, self-awareness, and supportive strategies to sustain positive changes and promote overall well-being. By incorporating healthy lifestyle habits, mindful eating practices, continued education, and regular health check-ups into your daily routine, you can cultivate a lasting foundation for optimal health and vitality. Remember that progress may be gradual, and setbacks are a natural part of the journey, so be patient, compassionate, and persistent in your efforts to prioritize your health and well-being.

BONUS: SOME HERBAL REMEDIES FOR HEALTH & WELLNESS

Ginseng:

Definition: Ginseng refers to several species of perennial plants belonging to the Panax genus, including Panax ginseng (Asian ginseng) and Panax quinquefolius (American ginseng). Ginseng has been used for centuries in traditional medicine, particularly in East Asia, for its potential health benefits.

Ingredients: Ginseng root contains various bioactive compounds, including ginsenosides, polysaccharides, and peptides. These compounds are believed to contribute to the herb's medicinal properties, including its potential as an adaptogen, immune enhancer, and cognitive booster.

How to Prepare: Ginseng is typically consumed as a powdered root, herbal tea, tincture, or in supplement form (such as capsules or tablets). To make tea, dried ginseng root slices are simmered in water for several minutes before being strained and consumed.

Dosage: The appropriate dosage of ginseng can vary depending on factors such as age, health status, and the specific preparation being used. It's important to follow the recommended dosage on the product label or consult with a qualified herbalist or healthcare professional for personalized guidance.

How to Use: Ginseng powder, tea, tincture, or supplements are typically taken orally. It's often used to support energy levels, enhance cognitive function, and promote overall well-being.

Side Effects: Ginseng is generally considered safe for most people when used in moderate amounts. However, some individuals may experience mild side effects such as insomnia, gastrointestinal upset, or headaches. It may also interact with certain medications or have adverse effects in individuals with certain health conditions, such as high blood pressure or diabetes. Pregnant or breastfeeding individuals should consult with a healthcare professional before using ginseng supplements. It's important to use ginseng under the guidance of a healthcare professional and to discontinue use if any adverse effects occur.

Goldenseal:

Definition: Goldenseal, scientifically known as Hydrastis canadensis, is a perennial herb native to North America. It has a long history of use in traditional Native American medicine and later in folk medicine for its potential health benefits.

Ingredients: Goldenseal root contains various bioactive compounds, including alkaloids (such as berberine and hydrastine), flavonoids, and volatile oils. These compounds are believed to contribute to the herb's medicinal properties, including its potential as an antimicrobial, anti-inflammatory, and immune enhancer.

How to Prepare: Goldenseal is typically consumed as an herbal tea, tincture, or in supplement form (such as capsules or tablets). To make tea, dried goldenseal root or leaves are steeped in hot water for several minutes before being strained and consumed.

Dosage: The appropriate dosage of goldenseal can vary depending on factors such as age, health status, and the specific preparation being used. It's important to follow the recommended dosage on the product label or consult with a qualified herbalist or healthcare professional for personalized guidance.

How to Use: Goldenseal tea, tincture, or supplements are typically taken orally. It's often used to support immune function, promote digestive health, and soothe inflammation.

Side Effects: Goldenseal is generally considered safe for most people when used in moderate amounts. However, some individuals may experience mild side effects such as gastrointestinal upset or allergic reactions. It may also interact with certain medications or have adverse effects in individuals with certain health conditions, such as high blood pressure or pregnancy. It's important to use goldenseal under the guidance of a healthcare professional and to discontinue use if any adverse effects occur.

Hops:

Definition: Hops, scientifically known as Humulus lupulus, is a perennial climbing vine native to Europe, Asia, and North America. It is primarily known for its use in brewing beer but has also been used historically in traditional medicine for its potential health benefits.

Ingredients: Hops flowers contain various bioactive compounds, including bitter acids (such as humulone and lupulone), essential oils, flavonoids, and polyphenols. These compounds are believed to contribute to the herb's medicinal properties, including its potential as a sedative, relaxant, and digestive aid.

How to Prepare: Hops is typically consumed as an herbal tea, tincture, or in supplement form (such as capsules or tablets). To make tea, dried hops flowers are steeped in hot water for several minutes before being strained and consumed.

Dosage: The appropriate dosage of hops can vary depending on factors such as age, health status, and the specific preparation being used. It's important to follow the recommended dosage on the product label or consult with a qualified herbalist or healthcare professional for personalized guidance.

How to Use: Hops tea, tincture, or supplements are typically taken orally. It's often used to promote relaxation, relieve anxiety, and support sleep.

Side Effects: Hops is generally considered safe for most people when used in moderate amounts. However, some individuals may experience mild side effects such as drowsiness, gastrointestinal upset, or allergic reactions. It may also interact with certain medications or have adverse effects in individuals with certain health conditions, such as depression or hormone-sensitive conditions. It's important to use hops under the guidance of a healthcare professional and to discontinue use if any adverse effects occur.

Bio Ferro Tonic:

Definition: Bio Ferro Tonic is a dietary supplement primarily composed of herbs and minerals. It's often marketed as a natural way to support overall health, particularly by promoting blood health and circulation.

Ingredients: Typical ingredients in Bio Ferro Tonic may include a blend of herbs such as burdock root, yellow dock root, sarsaparilla root, and cascara sagrada bark, along with minerals like iron and potassium phosphate.

How to Prepare: Bio Ferro Tonic usually comes in liquid form and is typically taken orally. It's important to follow the instructions on the product label for dosage and administration.

Dosage: The dosage can vary depending on the specific product and individual needs. It's crucial to consult with a healthcare professional or follow the recommended dosage on the product label to avoid potential side effects.

How to Use: Bio Ferro Tonic is often taken by adding the recommended dosage to water or juice and consuming it orally. It's important to shake the bottle well before use and store it according to the manufacturer's instructions.

Side Effects: While Bio Ferro Tonic is generally considered safe when used as directed, some individuals may experience side effects such as digestive discomfort, allergic reactions, or interactions with medications. It's essential to consult with a healthcare provider before starting any new supplement regimen, especially if you have underlying health conditions or are taking medications.

Bladderwrack:

Definition: Bladderwrack is a type of seaweed or marine algae commonly used in traditional medicine and as a dietary supplement. It's known for its potential health benefits, particularly related to thyroid health and weight management.

Ingredients: Bladderwrack contains various nutrients, including iodine, vitamins, minerals, and antioxidants. The primary active components are iodine and fucoidan, a type of carbohydrate found in brown seaweeds.

How to Prepare: Bladderwrack supplements are available in various forms, including capsules, powders, and liquid extracts. They can be taken orally with water or added to smoothies and other beverages.

Dosage: The appropriate dosage of bladderwrack can vary based on factors such as age, health status, and the specific product being used. It's essential to follow the recommended dosage on the product label or consult with a healthcare professional for personalized guidance.

How to Use: Bladderwrack supplements are typically taken orally, either with water or mixed into food or beverages. It's important to follow the instructions on the product label and avoid exceeding the recommended dosage.

Side Effects: While bladderwrack is generally considered safe for most people when used in moderation, excessive intake of iodine from bladderwrack supplements can cause thyroid dysfunction and other adverse effects. Individuals with thyroid disorders, iodine sensitivity, or certain medical conditions should exercise caution and consult with a healthcare provider before using bladderwrack supplements. Common side effects may include digestive upset, allergic reactions, or interactions with medications.

Blood Purifier:

Definition: Blood purifiers are herbal remedies or dietary supplements believed to cleanse or detoxify the blood, often promoting overall health and well-being. They are thought to support the body's natural detoxification processes and improve blood circulation.

Ingredients: Blood purifiers may contain a variety of herbs and botanical extracts known for their purported cleansing and detoxifying properties. Common ingredients include burdock root, red clover, dandelion root, and yellow dock root, among others.

How to Prepare: Blood purifiers are typically available in various forms, including capsules, tablets, powders, and liquid extracts. They are usually taken orally with water or juice, following the recommended dosage on the product label.

Dosage: The dosage of blood purifiers can vary depending on the specific product and individual needs. It's important to adhere to the recommended dosage on the product label or consult with a healthcare professional for personalized guidance.

How to Use: Blood purifiers are typically taken orally, either with water or mixed into beverages. They are often used as part of a detoxification regimen or to support overall health and vitality.

Side Effects: While blood purifiers are generally considered safe for most people when used as directed, some individuals may experience side effects such as digestive discomfort, allergic reactions, or interactions with medications. It's important to consult with a healthcare provider before starting any new supplement regimen, especially if you have underlying health conditions or are taking medications.

Blue Vervain:

Definition: Blue vervain, also known as Verbena hastata, is a perennial herb native to North America. It has been used in traditional medicine for centuries to treat various ailments, including anxiety, insomnia, and digestive issues.

Ingredients: Blue vervain contains several active compounds, including aucubin, verbenalin, and volatile oils. These compounds are believed to contribute to the herb's medicinal properties.

How to Prepare: Blue vervain is typically consumed as a tea or tincture. To make tea, dried blue vervain leaves and flowers are steeped in hot water for several minutes before being strained and consumed. Tinctures are prepared by steeping the herb in alcohol or vinegar to extract its active compounds.

Dosage: The appropriate dosage of blue vervain can vary depending on factors such as age, health status, and the specific preparation being used. It's important to follow the recommended dosage on the product label or consult with a qualified herbalist or healthcare professional for personalized guidance.

How to Use: Blue vervain tea or tincture is typically taken orally. It can be consumed on its own or mixed with honey or other herbal teas for added flavor.

Side Effects: While blue vervain is generally considered safe for most people when used in moderation, excessive intake may cause digestive upset or allergic reactions in some individuals. Pregnant or breastfeeding women should avoid blue vervain due to its potential to stimulate uterine contractions. As with any herbal remedy, it's important to consult with a healthcare provider before using blue vervain, especially if you have underlying health conditions or are taking medications.

Bromide Plus Powder:

Definition: Bromide Plus Powder is a dietary supplement formulated to support thyroid health and promote overall well-being. It typically contains a blend of herbs and minerals that are believed to have beneficial effects on thyroid function.

Ingredients: Bromide Plus Powder often contains a combination of herbs such as bladderwrack, sea moss, and burdock root, along with minerals like iodine and potassium phosphate. These ingredients are thought to support thyroid function and maintain optimal iodine levels in the body.

How to Prepare: Bromide Plus Powder is usually mixed with water or juice to create a drinkable solution. It's important to follow the instructions on the product label for dosage and preparation.

Dosage: The dosage of Bromide Plus Powder can vary depending on the specific product and individual needs. It's crucial to consult with a healthcare professional or follow the recommended dosage on the product label to avoid potential side effects.

How to Use: Bromide Plus Powder is typically taken orally by mixing the recommended dosage with water or juice. It's important to shake or stir the mixture well before consuming it to ensure even distribution of the ingredients.

Side Effects: While Bromide Plus Powder is generally considered safe when used as directed, some individuals may experience side effects such as digestive discomfort or allergic reactions to certain ingredients. It's essential to consult with a healthcare provider before starting any new supplement regimen, especially if you have underlying health conditions or are taking medications.

Bugleweed:

Definition: Bugleweed, also known as Lycopusvirginicus, is a perennial herb native to North America and Europe. It has been used in traditional medicine to treat various conditions, including hyperthyroidism, anxiety, and insomnia.

Ingredients: Bugleweed contains several active compounds, including lithospermic acid, phenolic acids, and flavonoids. These compounds are believed to contribute to the herb's medicinal properties, particularly its ability to regulate thyroid function.

How to Prepare: Bugleweed is commonly consumed as a tea or tincture. To make tea, dried bugleweed leaves and flowers are steeped in hot water for several minutes before being strained and consumed. Tinctures are prepared by steeping the herb in alcohol or vinegar to extract its active compounds.

Dosage: The appropriate dosage of bugleweed can vary depending on factors such as age, health status, and the specific preparation being used. It's important to follow the recommended dosage on the product label or consult with a qualified herbalist or healthcare professional for personalized guidance.

How to Use: Bugleweed tea or tincture is typically taken orally. It can be consumed on its own or mixed with honey or other herbal teas for added flavor.

Side Effects: While bugleweed is generally considered safe for most people when used in moderation, excessive intake may cause digestive upset or allergic reactions in some individuals. Pregnant or breastfeeding women should avoid bugleweed due to its potential to stimulate uterine contractions. As with any herbal remedy, it's important to consult with a healthcare provider before using bugleweed, especially if you have underlying health conditions or are taking medications.

Burdock:

Definition: Burdock, scientifically known as Arctium lappa, is a biennial plant native to Europe and Asia but now found worldwide. It's part of the Asteraceae family and has been used for centuries in traditional medicine and culinary practices.

Ingredients: Burdock contains various nutrients, including carbohydrates, fiber, vitamins (such as vitamin B6, folate, and vitamin C), and minerals (including potassium, magnesium, and manganese). It also contains active compounds such as polyphenols and volatile oils.

How to Prepare: Burdock can be prepared and consumed in various ways. The roots, leaves, and seeds are all utilized for different purposes. The root is commonly used in cooking, herbal teas, tinctures, and supplements, while the leaves and seeds are sometimes used in herbal preparations.

Dosage: The appropriate dosage of burdock root can vary depending on the specific form and intended use. For culinary purposes, there are no strict dosage guidelines, but for supplements or herbal remedies, it's essential to follow the recommended dosage on the product label or consult with a healthcare professional.

How to Use: Burdock root can be used in cooking by peeling, slicing, and adding it to soups, stews, stir-fries, or salads. It can also be brewed into a tea or used to make tinctures or extracts for medicinal purposes. Some people may also take burdock root supplements in capsule or powder form.

Side Effects: While burdock is generally considered safe for most people when consumed in moderate amounts, some individuals may experience allergic reactions or digestive upset. Additionally, burdock may interact with certain medications or have adverse effects in individuals with certain health conditions, such as diabetes or allergies to plants in the Asteraceae family. It's important to consult with a healthcare provider before using burdock, especially if you have underlying health conditions or are taking medications.

Cascara Sagrada:

Definition: Cascara Sagrada, scientifically known as Rhamnus purshiana, is a species of buckthorn native to western North America. It has been used traditionally as a laxative and to promote bowel regularity.

Ingredients: The primary active ingredients in cascara sagrada are anthraquinone glycosides, particularly cascarosides A and B. These compounds stimulate peristalsis in the colon, leading to increased bowel movements.

How to Prepare: Cascara sagrada is typically prepared as an herbal tea, tincture, or capsule. To make tea, dried cascara sagrada bark is steeped in hot water for several minutes before being strained and consumed. Tinctures are prepared by steeping the bark in alcohol to extract its active compounds.

Dosage: The appropriate dosage of cascara sagrada can vary depending on the specific preparation and intended use. It's important to follow the recommended dosage on the product label or consult with a healthcare professional for personalized guidance.

How to Use: Cascara sagrada tea or tincture is typically taken orally. It's important to start with a low dose and gradually increase if needed to avoid potential side effects such as cramping or diarrhea.

Side Effects: Cascara sagrada is considered safe for short-term use when used as directed. However, long-term or excessive use may lead to dependence, electrolyte imbalance, or dehydration. It may also interact with certain medications or have adverse effects in individuals with certain health conditions. It's important to use cascara sagrada under the guidance of a healthcare professional and to discontinue use if any adverse effects occur.

Cell Food:

Definition: Cell Food is a dietary supplement marketed as a highly oxygenating and alkalizing formula. It's claimed to support overall health and vitality by providing essential nutrients and oxygen to the cells.

Ingredients: The exact ingredients of Cell Food can vary depending on the brand, but it typically contains a proprietary blend of minerals, enzymes, electrolytes, and trace elements. Some common ingredients may include purified water, dissolved oxygen, seawater extract, and plant-based enzymes.

How to Prepare: Cell Food is usually available in liquid form and is typically taken orally. It can be consumed directly or diluted in water or juice before consumption.

Dosage: The dosage of Cell Food can vary depending on the specific product and individual needs. It's important to follow the recommended dosage on the product label or consult with a healthcare professional for personalized guidance.

How to Use: Cell Food is typically taken orally, either directly or mixed into water or juice. It's important to shake the bottle well before use and to store it according to the manufacturer's instructions.

Side Effects: Cell Food is generally considered safe for most people when used as directed. However, some individuals may experience mild digestive upset or allergic reactions to certain ingredients. It's essential to consult with a healthcare provider before starting any new supplement regimen, especially if you have underlying health conditions or are taking medications.

Chaparral:

Definition: Chaparral, scientifically known as Larrea tridentata, is a shrub native to the southwestern United States and northern Mexico. It has been used for centuries by Native American tribes for its medicinal properties and is commonly used in herbal medicine today.

Ingredients: Chaparral contains several bioactive compounds, including nordihydroguaiaretic acid (NDGA), flavonoids, lignans, and volatile oils. NDGA is believed to be the primary active compound responsible for many of chaparral's therapeutic effects.

How to Prepare: Chaparral can be prepared and consumed in various forms, including teas, tinctures, capsules, and topical preparations. To make tea, dried chaparral leaves are steeped in hot water for several minutes before being strained and consumed. Tinctures are prepared by steeping the herb in alcohol or vinegar to extract its active compounds.

Dosage: The appropriate dosage of chaparral can vary depending on the specific form and intended use. It's important to follow the recommended dosage on the product label or consult with a healthcare professional for personalized guidance.

How to Use: Chaparral tea or tincture is typically taken orally. It can also be applied topically to the skin for certain conditions. It's important to use chaparral products as directed and to discontinue use if any adverse effects occur.

Side Effects: Chaparral is generally considered safe for most people when used in moderate amounts. However, excessive intake or prolonged use may lead to liver toxicity or other adverse effects. It may also interact with certain medications or have adverse effects in individuals with certain health conditions. It's important to use chaparral under the guidance of a healthcare professional and to discontinue use if any adverse effects occur.

Cocolmeca:

Definition: Cocolmeca, also known as Smilax ornata or sarsaparilla, is a flowering vine native to Mexico and Central America. It has been used traditionally in Mexican and Central American folk medicine for its purported medicinal properties.

Ingredients: Cocolmeca contains various bioactive compounds, including saponins, flavonoids, and plant sterols. These compounds are believed to contribute to the herb's medicinal properties, including its potential as a diuretic, blood purifier, and anti-inflammatory agent.

How to Prepare: Cocolmeca is commonly prepared and consumed as an herbal tea or decoction. To make tea, dried cocolmeca roots or leaves are steeped in hot water for several minutes before being strained and consumed. Decoctions involve boiling the roots or leaves in water to extract their active compounds.

Dosage: The appropriate dosage of cocolmeca can vary depending on factors such as age, health status, and the specific preparation being used. It's important to follow the recommended dosage on the product label or consult with a qualified herbalist or healthcare professional for personalized guidance.

How to Use: Cocolmeca tea or decoction is typically taken orally. It can also be used topically for certain skin conditions. It's important to use cocolmeca products as directed and to discontinue use if any adverse effects occur.

Side Effects: Cocolmeca is generally considered safe for most people when used in moderate amounts. However, excessive intake may lead to digestive upset or other adverse effects. It may also interact with certain medications or have adverse effects in individuals with certain health conditions. It's important to use cocolmeca under the guidance of a healthcare professional and to discontinue use if any adverse effects occur.

Contribo:

Definition: Contribo, also known as Aristolochiatrilobata, is a vine native to the Caribbean and Central America. It has been used traditionally in folk medicine for various purposes, including as a remedy for digestive issues, inflammation, and pain relief.

Ingredients: Contribo contains several bioactive compounds, including aristolochic acids, flavonoids, and alkaloids. These compounds are believed to contribute to the herb's medicinal properties, including its potential as an anti-inflammatory and analgesic agent.

How to Prepare: Contribo is typically prepared and consumed as an herbal tea or decoction. To make tea, dried contribo leaves or stems are steeped in hot water for several minutes before being strained and consumed. Decoctions involve boiling the leaves or stems in water to extract their active compounds.

Dosage: The appropriate dosage of contribo can vary depending on factors such as age, health status, and the specific preparation being used. It's important to follow the recommended dosage on the product label or consult with a qualified herbalist or healthcare professional for personalized guidance.

How to Use: Contribo tea or decoction is typically taken orally. It's important to use contribo products as directed and to discontinue use if any adverse effects occur.

Side Effects: Contribo contains aristolochic acids, which have been associated with serious adverse effects, including kidney damage and cancer. Due to these safety concerns, the use of contribo is highly discouraged, and it's important to avoid products containing aristolochic acids. Individuals should seek alternative remedies for their health needs.

Dandelion Root:

Definition: Dandelion, scientifically known as Taraxacum officinale, is a common flowering plant found worldwide. While often considered a pesky weed, dandelion has a long history of use in traditional medicine for its various health benefits.

Ingredients: Dandelion root contains several bioactive compounds, including sesquiterpene lactones, triterpenes, flavonoids, and polysaccharides. These compounds are believed to contribute to the herb's medicinal properties, including its potential as a diuretic, digestive aid, and liver tonic.

How to Prepare: Dandelion root can be prepared and consumed in various forms, including teas, tinctures, capsules, and extracts. To make tea, dried dandelion root is steeped in hot water for several minutes before being strained and consumed. Tinctures are prepared by steeping the root in alcohol or vinegar to extract its active compounds.

Dosage: The appropriate dosage of dandelion root can vary depending on factors such as age, health status, and the specific preparation being used. It's important to follow the recommended dosage on the product label or consult with a qualified herbalist or healthcare professional for personalized guidance.

How to Use: Dandelion root tea, tincture, or capsules are typically taken orally. It's important to use dandelion root products as directed and to discontinue use if any adverse effects occur.

Side Effects: Dandelion root is generally considered safe for most people when used in moderate amounts. However, some individuals may experience allergic reactions or digestive upset. It may also interact with certain medications or have adverse effects in individuals with certain health conditions. It's important to use dandelion root under the guidance of a healthcare professional and to discontinue use if any adverse effects occur.

Herban Iron:

Definition: Herban Iron is a dietary supplement designed to provide an easily absorbable form of iron to support healthy iron levels in the body. It's particularly beneficial for individuals with iron deficiency or anemia.

Ingredients: Herban Iron typically contains iron in the form of ferrous bisglycinate, which is a highly bioavailable and gentle form of iron that is less likely to cause digestive upset or constipation compared to other forms of iron. It may also contain other ingredients such as vitamin C to enhance iron absorption.

How to Prepare: Herban Iron is usually available in capsule or liquid form. Capsules are taken orally with water, while liquid forms may be mixed with water or juice before consumption. It's important to follow the recommended dosage on the product label.

Dosage: The appropriate dosage of Herban Iron depends on factors such as age, gender, and the severity of iron deficiency. It's important to consult with a healthcare professional to determine the correct dosage for individual needs.

How to Use: Herban Iron capsules are typically taken orally with water, while liquid forms may be mixed with water or juice before consumption. It's important to take Herban Iron as directed and to avoid taking it with dairy products, antacids, or other substances that may interfere with iron absorption.

Side Effects: While Herban Iron is generally considered safe for most people when used as directed, some individuals may experience mild side effects such as gastrointestinal discomfort or constipation. It's important to consult with a healthcare professional before starting any new supplement regimen, especially if you have underlying health conditions or are taking medications.

Hydrangea:

Definition: Hydrangea, scientifically known as Hydrangea arborescens, is a flowering shrub native to North America. It has been used traditionally in herbal medicine for its potential diuretic and anti-inflammatory properties.

Ingredients: Hydrangea contains several bioactive compounds, including saponins, flavonoids, and glycosides. These compounds are believed to contribute to the herb's medicinal properties, including its potential as a diuretic, kidney tonic, and anti-inflammatory agent.

How to Prepare: Hydrangea root is typically prepared and consumed as an herbal tea or tincture. To make tea, dried hydrangea root is steeped in hot water for several minutes before being strained and consumed. Tinctures are prepared by steeping the root in alcohol or vinegar to extract its active compounds.

Dosage: The appropriate dosage of hydrangea can vary depending on factors such as age, health status, and the specific preparation being used. It's important to follow the recommended dosage on the product label or consult with a qualified herbalist or healthcare professional for personalized guidance.

How to Use: Hydrangea tea or tincture is typically taken orally. It's important to use hydrangea products as directed and to discontinue use if any adverse effects occur.

Side Effects: Hydrangea is generally considered safe for most people when used in moderate amounts. However, some individuals may experience digestive upset or allergic reactions. It may also interact with certain medications or have adverse effects in individuals with certain health conditions. It's important to use hydrangea under the guidance of a healthcare professional and to discontinue use if any adverse effects occur.

Irish Moss:

Definition: Irish Moss, scientifically known as Chondrus crispus, is a species of red algae or seaweed native to the Atlantic coastlines of Europe and North America. It has been used for centuries in traditional Irish and Scottish cuisine, as well as in herbal medicine.

Ingredients: Irish Moss is rich in various nutrients, including iodine, sulfur compounds, vitamins (such as vitamin A, vitamin K, and vitamin B12), minerals (including calcium, magnesium, potassium, and sodium), and polysaccharides (such as carrageenan). These nutrients are believed to contribute to the herb's potential health benefits.

How to Prepare: Irish Moss is typically prepared by soaking it in water to rehydrate and soften it before use. It can be added to soups, stews, smoothies, desserts, and other dishes as a thickening agent or nutritional supplement.

Dosage: The appropriate dosage of Irish Moss can vary depending on factors such as age, health status, and the specific preparation being used. It's important to follow recipes or guidelines for culinary use and to consult with a healthcare professional for guidance on using Irish Moss as a dietary supplement.

How to Use: Irish Moss can be used in culinary applications to add thickness and nutritional value to dishes. It can also be consumed as a dietary supplement in the form of capsules, powders, or extracts.

Side Effects: Irish Moss is generally considered safe for most people when consumed in moderate amounts as part of a balanced diet. However, some individuals may be allergic to seaweed or carrageenan, a compound found in Irish Moss that is used as a food additive. It's important to discontinue use if any adverse effects occur and to consult with a healthcare professional if you have any concerns.

Irish Sea Moss:

Definition: Irish Sea Moss is a term often used interchangeably with Irish Moss, referring to the same species of red algae, Chondrus crispus. It's harvested from the rocky shores of the Atlantic coastlines of Europe and North America.

Ingredients: Irish Sea Moss shares the same nutritional profile as Irish Moss, containing iodine, vitamins, minerals, and polysaccharides. It's valued for its potential health benefits, including supporting thyroid function, boosting immune health, and promoting digestion.

How to Prepare: Irish Sea Moss is prepared in the same way as Irish Moss, by soaking it in water to rehydrate and soften it before use. It can be used in culinary applications or consumed as a dietary supplement.

Dosage: The dosage of Irish Sea Moss depends on the form and intended use. As a dietary supplement, it's important to follow the recommended dosage on the product label or consult with a healthcare professional for personalized guidance.

How to Use: Irish Sea Moss can be used in various culinary applications, including soups, smoothies, desserts, and sauces. It can also be consumed as a dietary supplement in the form of capsules, powders, or extracts.

Side Effects: Similar to Irish Moss, Irish Sea Moss is generally considered safe for most people when consumed in moderate amounts. However, individuals with seaweed allergies or sensitivities to carrageenan should exercise caution. It's important to discontinue use if any adverse effects occur and to consult with a healthcare professional if you have any concerns.

Lymphalin:

Definition: Lymphalin is a herbal supplement formulated to support lymphatic system health. The lymphatic system plays a crucial role in immune function and waste removal in the body, and Lymphalin is designed to promote its proper function.

Ingredients: Lymphalin typically contains a blend of herbs and botanical extracts known for their traditional use in supporting lymphatic system health. Common ingredients may include cleavers, red clover, echinacea, burdock root, and calendula, among others.

How to Prepare: Lymphalin is usually available in capsule or liquid form. Capsules are taken orally with water, while liquid forms may be mixed with water or juice before consumption. It's important to follow the recommended dosage on the product label.

Dosage: The appropriate dosage of Lymphalin can vary depending on the specific product and individual needs. It's important to follow the recommended dosage on the product label or consult with a healthcare professional for personalized guidance.

How to Use: Lymphalin capsules are typically taken orally with water, while liquid forms may be mixed with water or juice before consumption. It's often recommended to take Lymphalin on an empty stomach for optimal absorption.

Side Effects: Lymphalin is generally considered safe for most people when used as directed. However, some individuals may experience mild side effects such as gastrointestinal discomfort or allergic reactions to certain ingredients. It's important to consult with a healthcare provider before starting any new supplement regimen, especially if you have underlying health conditions or are taking medications.

Green Food Plus:

Definition: Green Food Plus is a dietary supplement formulated to provide a concentrated source of nutrients derived from various green plants. It's designed to support overall health and well-being by delivering essential vitamins, minerals, antioxidants, and phytonutrients.

Ingredients: Green Food Plus typically contains a blend of powdered green vegetables, grasses, algae, and other plant-based ingredients. Common ingredients may include wheatgrass, barley grass, spirulina, chlorella, alfalfa, kale, spinach, and broccoli, among others.

How to Prepare: Green Food Plus is usually available in powder form and can be mixed with water, juice, or smoothies. It's important to follow the recommended dosage on the product label and to consume it as part of a balanced diet.

Dosage: The appropriate dosage of Green Food Plus can vary depending on the specific product and individual needs. It's important to follow the recommended dosage on the product label or consult with a healthcare professional for personalized guidance.

How to Use: Green Food Plus powder is typically mixed with water, juice, or smoothies and consumed orally. It's often taken once or twice daily, preferably with meals, to maximize nutrient absorption.

Side Effects: Green Food Plus is generally considered safe for most people when used as directed. However, some individuals may experience digestive upset or allergic reactions to certain ingredients. It's important to consult with a healthcare provider before starting any new supplement regimen, especially if you have underlying health conditions or are taking medications.

Guaco:

Definition: Guaco, also known as Mikania cordata or Mikania glomerata, is a medicinal plant native to Central and South America. It has a long history of use in traditional medicine for its potential therapeutic properties.

Ingredients: Guaco contains several bioactive compounds, including coumarins, flavonoids, tannins, and saponins. These compounds are believed to contribute to the herb's medicinal properties, including its potential as an expectorant, anti-inflammatory, and antispasmodic agent.

How to Prepare: Guaco is typically prepared and consumed as an herbal tea or infusion. To make tea, dried guaco leaves are steeped in hot water for several minutes before being strained and consumed.

Dosage: The appropriate dosage of guaco can vary depending on factors such as age, health status, and the specific preparation being used. It's important to follow the recommended dosage on the product label or consult with a qualified herbalist or healthcare professional for personalized guidance.

How to Use: Guaco tea is typically taken orally. It can be consumed on its own or mixed with honey or other herbal teas for added flavor.

Side Effects: Guaco is generally considered safe for most people when used in moderate amounts. However, some individuals may experience allergic reactions or digestive upset. It may also interact with certain medications or have adverse effects in individuals with certain health conditions. It's important to use guaco under the guidance of a healthcare professional and to discontinue use if any adverse effects occur.

Kelp:

Definition: Kelp refers to several species of large brown algae belonging to the Laminariales order. It is commonly found in underwater forests along rocky coastlines around the world. Kelp has been used for centuries in various cultures, particularly in East Asia, for its nutritional and medicinal properties.

Ingredients: Kelp is rich in various nutrients, including iodine, vitamins (such as vitamin K, vitamin C, and B vitamins), minerals (including calcium, magnesium, and potassium), antioxidants, and fiber. These nutrients are believed to contribute to the seaweed's potential health benefits, including its role in thyroid function, bone health, and immune support.

How to Prepare: Kelp is typically consumed dried, powdered, or in supplement form (such as capsules or tablets). It can also be used in cooking, particularly in soups, salads, and stir-fries. Kelp supplements are available in various forms, including powdered extracts, tablets, and liquid extracts.

Dosage: The appropriate dosage of kelp can vary depending on factors such as age, health status, and the specific preparation being used. It's important to follow the recommended dosage on the product label or consult with a qualified healthcare professional for personalized guidance.

How to Use: Kelp supplements are typically taken orally with water. They can be consumed as part of a daily nutritional regimen to support overall health and well-being. Kelp can also be incorporated into recipes as a flavorful and nutritious ingredient.

Side Effects: While kelp is generally considered safe for most people when consumed in moderate amounts, excessive intake of iodine-rich foods or supplements, including kelp, can lead to thyroid dysfunction or iodine toxicity. Some individuals may also be allergic to seaweed and experience allergic reactions. Pregnant or breastfeeding individuals should consult with a healthcare professional before using kelp supplements. It's important to use kelp under the guidance of a healthcare professional and to discontinue use if any adverse effects occur.

Eucalyptus:

Definition: Eucalyptus refers to a genus of flowering trees and shrubs, primarily native to Australia but also found in other parts of the world. Eucalyptus essential oil, extracted from the leaves of certain species, has a long history of use in traditional medicine for its potential health benefits.

Ingredients: Eucalyptus essential oil contains various bioactive compounds, including eucalyptol (cineole), terpenes, and flavonoids. These compounds are believed to contribute to the oil's medicinal properties, including its potential as an expectorant, decongestant, antiseptic, and anti-inflammatory.

How to Prepare: Eucalyptus essential oil can be used in aromatherapy, diffused in the air, or diluted and applied topically to the skin. It can also be added to steam inhalations or chest rubs to help relieve respiratory symptoms.

Dosage: The appropriate dosage of eucalyptus essential oil can vary depending on factors such as age, health status, and the specific application being used. It's important to follow the recommended dosage on the product label or consult with a qualified aromatherapist or healthcare professional for personalized guidance.

How to Use: Eucalyptus essential oil can be used aromatically, topically, or internally, depending on the intended application. It's often used to alleviate respiratory congestion, soothe sore muscles, promote relaxation, and support overall well-being.

Side Effects: Eucalyptus essential oil is generally considered safe for most people when used appropriately. However, it can be toxic if ingested in large amounts and should not be applied directly to the skin without proper dilution. Some individuals may experience allergic reactions or respiratory irritation when exposed to eucalyptus oil. It's important to use eucalyptus oil with caution, especially around children and pets. Pregnant or breastfeeding individuals should consult with a healthcare professional before using eucalyptus oil. If any adverse effects occur, discontinue use and seek medical attention.

Feverfew:

Definition: Feverfew, scientifically known as Tanacetum parthenium, is a perennial herb native to Europe but also found in other parts of the world. It has a long history of use in traditional medicine, particularly in European folk medicine, for its potential health benefits.

Ingredients: Feverfew contains various bioactive compounds, including sesquiterpene lactones (such as parthenolide), flavonoids, and volatile oils. These compounds are believed to contribute to the herb's medicinal properties, including its potential as an anti-inflammatory, analgesic, and migraine prophylactic.

How to Prepare: Feverfew is typically consumed as an herbal tea, tincture, or in supplement form (such as capsules or tablets). To make tea, dried feverfew leaves and flowers are steeped in hot water for several minutes before being strained and consumed.

Dosage: The appropriate dosage of feverfew can vary depending on factors such as age, health status, and the specific preparation being used. It's important to follow the recommended dosage on the product label or consult with a qualified herbalist or healthcare professional for personalized guidance.

How to Use: Feverfew tea, tincture, or supplements are typically taken orally. It's often used to alleviate headaches, including migraines, and to support overall well-being.

Side Effects: Feverfew is generally considered safe for most people when used in moderate amounts. However, some individuals may experience mild side effects such as gastrointestinal upset or allergic reactions. It may also interact with certain medications or have adverse effects in individuals with certain health conditions, such as bleeding disorders or pregnancy. It's important to use feverfew under the guidance of a healthcare professional and to discontinue use if any adverse effects occur.

THE END